SKINNING THE CAT:

A BABY BOOMER'S GUIDE TO THE NEW RETIREE LIFESTYLES

by

Joan Fitting Scott

Copyright © 2006 by Joan Fitting Scott

All rights reserved. No part of this book shall be reproduced or transmitted in any form or by any means, electronic, mechanical, magnetic, photographic including photocopying, recording or by any information storage and retrieval system, without prior written permission of the publisher. No patent liability is assumed with respect to the use of the information contained herein. Although every precaution has been taken in the preparation of this book, the publisher and author assume no responsibility for errors or omissions. Neither is any liability assumed for damages resulting from the use of the information contained herein.

ISBN 0-7414-3358-3

Published by:

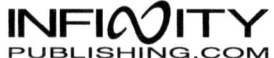

1094 New DeHaven Street, Suite 100
West Conshohocken, PA 19428-2713
Info@buybooksontheweb.com
www.buybooksontheweb.com
Toll-free (877) BUY BOOK
Local Phone (610) 941-9999
Fax (610) 941-9959

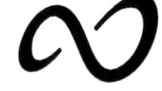

Printed in the United States of America

Printed on Recycled Paper

Published September 2006

TABLE OF CONTENTS

Introduction: A Different Way of Looking at Things i

Part One: Skinning the Cat: The Many Ways to Be Retired

Chapter 1: Continuing to Work 3
Chapter 2: Getting a New Job,
 Starting a New Business 9
Chapter 3: Working Part Time or Cyclically 15
Chapter 4: Not Working 19
Chapter 5: Volunteerism and Philanthropy 23
Chapter 6: Lifelong Learning 35
Chapter 7: Travel 39
Chapter 8: The Sabbatical 43

Part Two: Resources For Making the Decision

Chapter 9: Thinking It Through 49
Chapter 10: Retreats 51
Chapter 11: Coaches 55
Chapter 12: Self-Help Groups 59
Chapter 13: Company-Sponsored Pre-Retirement
 Workshops 61
Chapter 14: Final Thoughts 63

Suggested Reading 67
About the Author 69

ACKNOWLEDGMENTS

This book would not have come to fruition without the help of my supporters.

I would like to thank:

* My mother, my biggest cheerleader.
* My husband, for thoughtful reading of the manuscript.
* My kids, for being such good friends.
* Gene Zipperlen, for his professionalism in copy editing the manuscript.
* Alan Speaker, for research support.
* Carol Hendrix, a true friend and book marketing visionary.
* Olyve Abbott, a writer friend who always had time to help.
* Lucile Davis, Marilyn Komechak, Mary Keilly, Emily Williams, Joyce Miller and other Freelance Writers Network friends who offered advice and help.

INTRODUCTION:

A DIFFERENT WAY OF LOOKING AT THINGS

When Dad retired after working for the same company nearly all his adult life, he celebrated with a party and collected his gold watch. Then he bought a copy of *The New York Times*, found a comfortable spot on the deck of the family cabin and hunkered down. Or, he picked up his golf clubs and headed out to the links at his age-segregated retirement development. That was what you did in those days.

How times have changed!

A 2003 news release from the North Carolina Center for Creative Retirement says that by 2010, nearly 11 million Americans will have stepped away from their place of employment, headed for retirement. But today's about-to-be retirees are no doubt among America's 76 million baby boomers, those born between 1945 and 1963, who make up about a third of the American population. They have a vastly different notion of what retirement means than did Dad.

Increasingly, boomers, people with multidimensional lives and roles, will see retirement as a time to rewrite the rules and reinvent themselves. This generation, the largest in American history, will eschew the script Dad handed down, viewing the second half of life as a period of continued growth, not decline — a notion its predecessors might have thought a contradiction in terms.

Boomers will ask themselves why they should wait to do what they truly want to do. They might also question the idea that they should disengage from society and quit working, rejecting the notion of formal retirement as a mechanism for removing older people from the workplace. And boomers will seek to find meaning, rather than just busyness, in the time they have left, viewing their lives in those terms as opposed to counting the years since birth. Retirement, they will contend, grew out of a different demographic and cultural milieu than is operative today.

After all, these are the people who marched in the streets and explored sex, drugs and rock 'n' roll. Cookie-cutter solutions won't work for them, nor will they tolerate situations in which people deem them unproductive and irrelevant as they age. Rejecting isolated, age-segregated enclaves, people in this group will also choose adventure over the risk-averse safety that characterized their parents' retirement. They will see retirement not as the sad end of their active lives but as the beginning of a trip to exciting new destinations.

Boomers will trade in their green eyeshades for whisks or pick up a painter's palette instead of a calculator. Lawyers will become innkeepers and bureaucrats will take up acting.

Or maybe, like Nancy Smith (not her real name), who recently retired from her job at a major West Coast university, today's about-to-be retiree will scale the heights; Nancy climbed 10,547-foot Lassen Peak in the

Lassen Volcanic National Park in Northern California just three weeks after leaving her job in academia. An adventurer like Nancy, retiree Karen Milan of Fort Worth, Texas, enjoyed a trip to Morocco, but she savored even more the opportunity it afforded her to camp in the Sahara Desert.

And then there are fellow Texans like David and Barbara Burns. After Dave's retirement from a national railroad, Barb and Dave began teaching Texas history classes at a local community college.

Today's retirees will not only explore heretofore undeveloped skills and interests. They will also seek to deepen their connection to self, friends, family, the wider world and God. They might desire as well to leave some kind of legacy. That could mean establishing a family foundation, writing a family history or starting a lobbying initiative.

People in this generation will also live longer, healthier lives than any previous group, so they will have lots of time to explore life's options. Rather than having only enough time to regret, as may have been true of previous generations, boomers will have time to reinvent themselves. Statistics show that today's 50-year-old woman with no history of heart disease or cancer could live past 90, Rieva Lesonsky notes in *Start Your Own Business: The Only Start-Up Book You'll Ever Need*. When the Social Security retirement system began in 1935, Jeri Sedlar and Rick Miners say in *Don't Retire, Rewire: Five Steps to Fulfilling Work that Fuels Your Passion, Suits Your Personality, or Fills Your Pocket*, benefits started at age 65 whereas the average person lived to age 61. Things have changed since 1935!

And if they continue to work in one form or another — and many boomers may choose to, whether for self-fulfillment or, increasingly, to cover health-care and insurance costs and discretionary expenses — they'll have more money to fund that life exploration. The Retirement Confidence Survey, released in April 2004 by the Employee Benefit Research Institute and others, found that 68 percent of current workers expected to work for pay after retirement. A nationwide poll conducted by the John J. Heldrich Center for Workforce Development at Rutgers University produced similar results.

Lots of books cover the subject of planning for retirement. For the most part, they deal with its financial issues and pitfalls.

This book, by contrast, addresses the many options for spending our time in retirement, as opposed to the usual look, which focuses on how we spend our money. It assumes that retirement is a financial possibility. Putting financial issues aside for the moment, it helps readers think long and hard about how they would spend their time – all other things being equal. The "what I would do if I had all the money in the world" game allows untrammeled investigation of (perhaps hidden) life goals.

The book has two parts. In Part One, consecutive chapters profile options for retirement, including continuing work (As in not retiring? Yes, that's an option if you want to stay in the game); starting a new job or business; working part time or cyclically; or not working, for example, taking up golf, volunteerism or philanthropy, travel, going back to school, etc. A final chapter addresses an intermediate option, taking a sabbatical before returning to work again.

Part Two addresses where to find help in choosing among this panoply of retirement options. Coaches, classes, retreats and other resources can help the proactive boomer find his or her way through the maze. A suggested reading list concludes the book.

This is an amazing time. Boomers don't generally do the tough, back-breaking physical jobs of earlier generations, so they won't need a prolonged rest at retirement. Mandatory retirement, for most jobs, is all but a thing of the past. Medical breakthroughs and medications that postpone mental deterioration as well as a greater awareness of illness prevention mean that today's retirees can look forward to a lifespan that is likely to exceed Dad's.

What will they do with that gift of time? There is no "right" answer. As is the case with looking at modern art, all assessments have validity. The idea is to give oneself permission to explore the options for spending time as a retiree, to have fun ruminating, and then to choose wisely.

PART ONE:

SKINNING THE CAT: THE MANY WAYS TO BE RETIRED

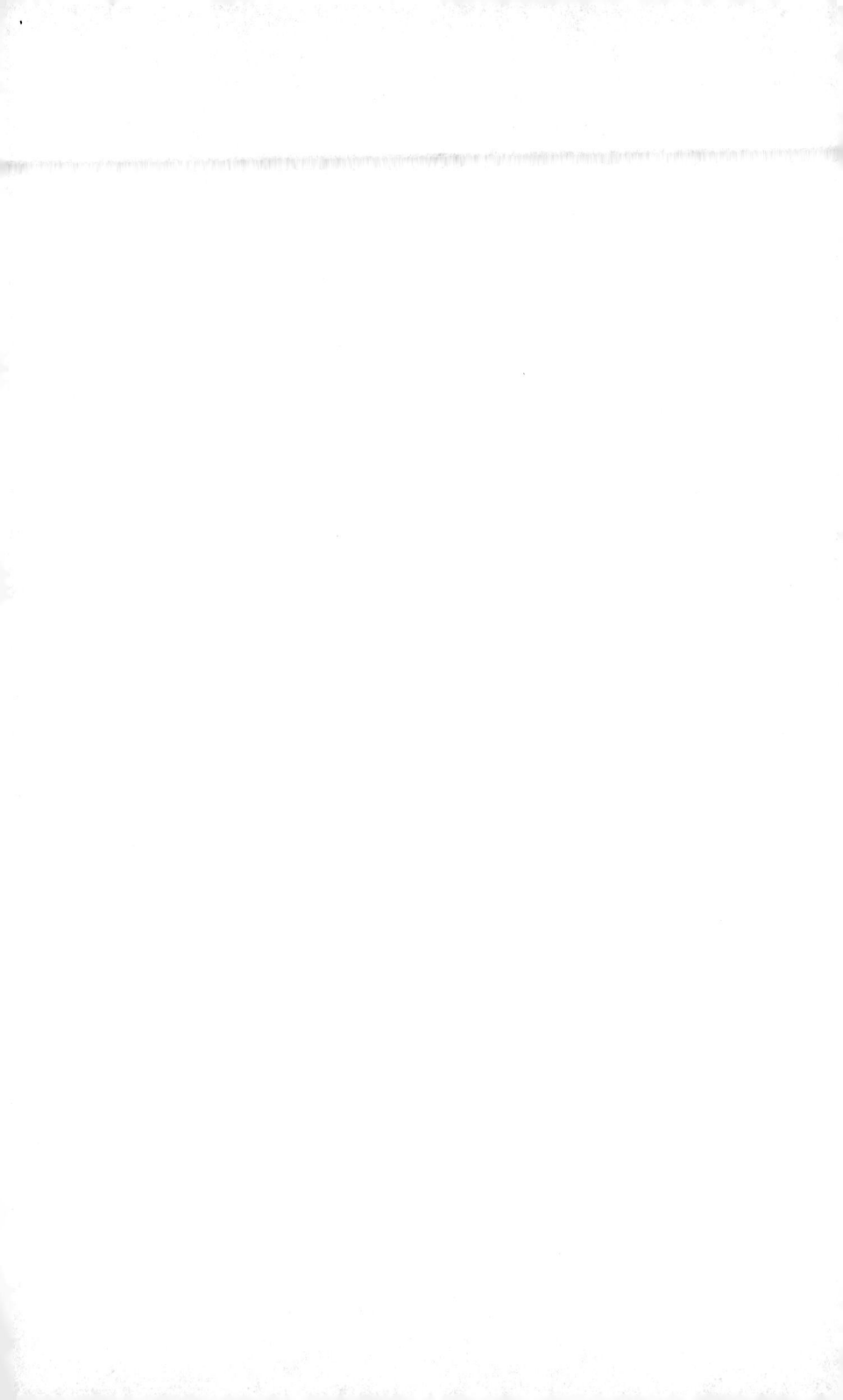

CHAPTER ONE:

CONTINUING TO WORK

How could continuing to work be a retirement option? After all, retiring means quitting work, doesn't it? Read on.

Stephen Clark retired at 58 and took up golf and fishing. He exercised. He bought a parcel of Florida sod and made plans to build a beach home. He took in the movie matinees with his wife, Paula.

This was retirement. And he hated it.

Though many people give up retirement for monetary reasons or can't retire in the first place for lack of funds, for others the decision either not to retire or to give up a false start at retirement has to do with missing being in the action.

After all, these people reason that they haven't seen any evidence suggesting that any age group has a monopoly on productivity. And according to a June 2005 *Business Week* article, "Old. Smart. Productive," the notion that older workers are less creative and flexible than their younger associates is largely a myth. So why shouldn't people in this age group be productively engaged if they want to be?

When Stephen Clark turned 60, he left his leisure behind and went back to work. He's once again a company president, reassuming a role he played earlier.

"I'm happy with my choice," he says. "I retired because I was burnt out, exhausted with my travel schedule. When I got rested, I missed the people and the activity. Now I'm back at it. I don't know how long my new career will last, but it's ideal for the moment. I retired too early the first time. Next time it'll be at the right time."

You might retire from a full-time job and immediately replace it with another full-time job. Or, like Stephen, you might retire and become bored and re-enter the work force.

Or you might consider retirement and then decide you'd miss being in the game. If the latter is the case, you could stay on the current job. Some options allow for continued work but at a more "retired" pace — one involving flexible schedules or transitions to retirement. In his book *Halftime: Changing Your Game Plan from Success to Significance*, Bob Buford addresses this in a chapter whose title says it all: "Staying in the Game but Adjusting the Plan." An example: At the University of Southern California, professors within two years of retirement may work half-time while retaining almost all benefits, says Janette Brown, Ed.D., executive director of the Emeriti Center.

At Sabre Holdings, flexible models "are an option," says Mike Haefner, senior vice president for human resources. "Our employees are encouraged to explore flex work arrangements with their supervisors and can job share, work part time or pursue other flex arrangements if it makes sense for the business."

Increasingly, America's companies, responding to demographic trends that suggest that a labor shortage is in the making, will feel pressure to devise these approaches to accommodate a burgeoning class of older workers. Data from the Bureau of Labor Statistics indicates that by 2012 the number of workers older than 55 will reach 31.1 million. And a March 2004 article in the *Harvard Business Review* said that by 2020 the U.S. work force will grow at a rate of about 0.2 percent annually. By that time workers 50 and older will make up as much as 80 percent of those employed in North America. Employers who want to get the most out of an aging pool of workers may soon need to embrace flexible work schedules, telecommuting and phased retirement, said William D. Novelli, chief executive of AARP, a large-membership group for older Americans, in remarks prepared for a June 2005 national symposium on the aging work force. And at the new Boston College Center on Aging and Work, a $3 million grant from the Alfred P. Sloan Foundation is funding a three-year study of how the American workplace is evolving to accommodate an older work force.

Phased retirement is an intriguing option. A January 2005 survey that Knowledge Networks conducted for AARP showed that two out of five workers age 50 or older were interested in the idea of phasing out of their careers by moving to part-time work in the same job. Nearly 80 percent of that group said the availability of such programs would encourage them to continue working longer.

Health-care providers in particular, eager to keep medical workers from retirement, offer well-developed programs, Kelly Greene reported in April 2005 in a *Wall Street Journal* "Encore" column. In fact, AARP has recognized several such programs, which allow employees to work part time while collecting full retirement and health benefits.

Another retirement alternative is "rehirement." The aforementioned *Business Week* article said that MITRE Corp., a Bedford, Massachusetts, research and development company, brought back retirees with valuable knowledge through a part-time on-call arrangement. Tom Heiserman, vice president for human resources at Lockheed Martin Aeronautics in Fort Worth, Texas, says his company occasionally uses a rehirement model as well, by bringing in former employees on a consulting or part-time basis. "Rehirement" is also an option at Sabre Holdings, Haefner says. And a Robert Half International survey found in early 2005 that 25 percent of the 150 executives responding planned to invite retirees and future retirees to be trainers and consultants.

Other arrangements also work. Deloitte Consulting LLC retains older workers through incentives like flextime and flexible work locations, the *Business Week* article said. And Borders Books has extended benefits including health-care and dental and vision plans to part-time workers. The company also allows flexible hours and part-of-the-year employment and store location switches that accommodate older workers dividing their time between winter and summer homes.

You may not want to retire abruptly but wish to move gradually in that direction. If you want to participate in phased retirement, project or contract jobs, or flextime or other flexible arrangements, transitioning your way to full leisure, it might be worthwhile to contact your company's human resources department to see if your company offers such arrangements.

The higher education and government sectors are currently the most common users of phased retirement programs, Sedlar and Miners say in *Don't Retire, Rewire: Five Steps to Fulfilling Work that Fuels Your Passion, Suits Your Personality, or Fills Your Pocket.* If the concept is foreign to your employer, you might use examples from these sectors; you might even propose a pilot program.

CHAPTER TWO:

GETTING A NEW JOB, STARTING A NEW BUSINESS

In the spring of 2005, investment giant Merrill Lynch rolled out the results of a study it conducted with Harris Interactive and Ken Dychtwald, Ph.D., author of *Age Wage, Age Power* and *The Power Years* and an authority on aging in America. The study, The Merrill Lynch New Retirement Survey: A Perspective From the Baby Boomer Generation, polled nearly 3,500 baby boomer respondents about their vision of retirement. Of the boomers who participated in the research, 56 percent of those who planned to continue working after officially retiring said they wanted to start new careers, and 13 percent said they wanted to start their own businesses. Far from slowing down, today's about-to-be-retireds are looking at ramping up in whole new lines of work, the study suggested.

Another recent study, conducted by the Rand Corp. for AARP, found that a growing number of older workers was buying or starting their own businesses. The percentage of 50-plus entrepreneurs is growing, the study found. In 2002, that age group accounted for 40.5 percent of the nation's self-employed, up from 37.6 percent in 1998. Self-employment across all other age groups, meanwhile, fell 6.8 percent.

A case in point: Michael and Marilyn Sakamoto of Sacramento, California. A July 2004 article in the *Sacramento Bee* described their choices. After Michael lost his software development job with Hewlett-Packard, the couple bought a bakery. They had lost faith in the whole idea of retirement after Michael's 23 years of service at the company ended, the article reported.

American corporations' penchant for downsizing has derailed lives and bred bitterness. Rather than be whipsawed, numbers of Americans have chosen to blaze their own employment trail and start their own businesses.

Others, their trust unshaken by adversity, do it less from necessity than desire. One of those people is Robert Goldberg, 57, of San Antonio, Texas. Robert is an attorney whose specialty was real estate law. Although he excelled at what he did in his previous career, he found real estate law contentious and adversarial. So he switched fields. Now he works in real estate development. "I like seeing my projects come to fruition and my clients happy," he says of his new venture. "I was good at the law, but it was never a great love of mine. Now I wake up every morning anxious to see the status of my current project."

After a long career in software engineering, Chandra Mouli decided he wanted to try something new. He had given some thought to the idea of opening an Indian restaurant and had seen a number that did a good business. Chandra liked the idea of starting a restaurant as a joint venture so he would have the flexibility to tend to his investments in his spare time.

Today Chandra has two restaurants, one in Milpitas, California, and one in Los Angeles. His U.S. partner is a longtime friend who has many years of business experience. His Indian partners are the owners of a long-established restaurant in India. Chandra's new business will focus on South Indian vegetarian dishes and a line of desserts. "Our chefs are trained by our Indian partners to produce the same authentic food we get back home and our products have brand recognition among Indians here in the United States. That's a real asset," he says.

Chandra enjoys his new career. "At first it was pretty demanding," he says. "But now we're up and running and things are going more smoothly. I like my new life. I have more control and more time to take care of my portfolio."

Marcia Traversaro and her husband John are the proud owners of Here for You, a personal services business based in the San Francisco Bay Area. Here for You helps people manage their busy lives by delivering goods to them and providing them services, Marcia says. "We buy people time," she says. Services include running errands, gift purchases and wrapping, and home organization and management. "We offer professional services that free our clients to do the things they find more rewarding and enjoyable," Marcia says.

Before she and her husband started their business, Marcia, a licensed clinical psychologist, worked in the human resources arena. She recently retired, as did her husband, a former battalion chief with the San Francisco Fire Department.

Upon retiring, the Traversaros bought a new home and embarked on an extensive remodeling. "The project we've undertaken is expensive," Marcia says, "and our business helps cover our costs. We're spending most of our time on our home and landscaping currently but will soon have more time to grow the business."

Marcia feels her retirement business allows them the opportunity to change from full-time jobs that pay expenses to work that more closely represents their passions.

"We do the things we enjoy and have options as to how much time and energy we're willing to spend on work. Our business also gives us a collaborative opportunity to meld our talents and inspirations in fun ways that expand our capabilities as well as our income."

Marcia and John have learned some good lessons since they began their new adventure. "As life experiences soften and mature our outlook, we realize it's not so much the attainment of the goal that's important, but the journey. We're still honing our skills in this game of life, but enjoying it so much more."

The Traversaros feel their business keeps them busy and in touch with the outside world. They were active in nonprofit causes during their working years and are used to a high level of activity. "Our business also satisfies our social needs," Marcia says.

If you're a corporate casualty, funding a dream or simply ready to try something new, don't be afraid of change. Do your research. Find a business you can buy, as did the Sakamotos, or move to a related but more satisfying field, as did Robert Goldberg. Or, like the Traversaros, invent a business that's your very own. You can also job-hunt your way to a new career. You might begin by surfing the 'Net. Try www.thephoenixlink.com, where you can post your resume if looking for a new job. Or have a look at www.yourencore.com, which recruits engineers, scientists and product developers. The AARP Web site, www.aarp.org, also lists employers looking for older workers, plus annual awards for the best employers for workers 50 or older.

CHAPTER THREE:

WORKING PART TIME OR CYCLICALLY

Of the boomers who participated in the Merrill Lynch study, better than half said they planned to work either part time or on a cyclical basis after officially retiring. Steve Mitchell, director of retirement marketing at Merrill Lynch in Plainsboro, New Jersey, says respondents who favored part-time or cyclical work did so because they thought interesting work would provide purpose and activity in their lives as well as extra funds.

"When they were asked why they wanted to work in the next phase, the boomers we talked to cited the need to keep mentally active rather than the need for the money," he says. The Cornell Retirement and Well-Being Study corroborates that finding, and an August 21, 2005, *Wall Street Journal* article reported that research showed that working seniors were happier than their nonworking counterparts.

Louis Armstrong of Arlington, Texas, exemplifies the point. He's retired from his job as a brewing team manager at Miller Brewing Co., where his responsibilities over the years included managing from six to 50 employees and budgets of more than $1 million. Louis now divides his time between volunteering and a part-time position as a golf pro.

Louis is happy to report to the links for his stint of 20 hours a week. "Upon retirement, I went to the local golf course and asked to be hired as a course marshal so I could play golf at a reduced rate," he says. "They hired me." During his time around the course Louis noticed deficiencies in management expertise; it was a new course with relatively inexperienced leadership. So he asked to play a larger role. "I acted as a trainer/consultant to a young man who was the golf professional at the time," he says. "I was asked to help him learn how to manage the business." However, it was decided that reorganization of the entire staff was necessary. Louis was then asked to act as interim manager while the course looked for a new general manager with experience in the golf business. "I worked that position for five months. Now I work in the pro shop three days a week and teach golf two days. I love the game and seeing others get enjoyment from it. This is the ideal retirement as far as I'm concerned."

Donna Dickinson also takes satisfaction in her less-than-full-time job. Dickinson, owner of Dickinson Equity Consulting, is a 60-something living in Half Moon Bay, California. She works as a consultant in equities compensation, managing and administering the finance, accounting, taxes, and securities rules and requirements for granting stock options to corporate employees.

Donna's consulting work is cyclical. She may join a company long enough to troubleshoot a problem, then take a break while awaiting another assignment. The rhythm of this arrangement suits her. She works very hard for a certain period and then has time for household chores and personal goals between gigs.

"I never want to retire," she says. "I want to stay in the game as long as I can. I'd be bored and lonely not working. And the extra cash helps with family expenses."

Boomers who enjoy the engagement of continuing to work might choose a part-time or cyclical schedule for two additional reasons: the demands involved in caring for their aging parents and a desire to spend time with their grandchildren. Attending to both sets of loved ones may require more free hours than a full-time job allows.

And boomers' changing priorities may dictate their work hours and cycle. This generation has purchased all the "stuff" it will ever need. More and more, boomers would rather buy experiences than things. They would prefer to travel and try new hobbies and interests on for size, as Ken Dychtwald, Ph.D., says in *Age Power: How the 21st Century Will Be Ruled by the New Old*. All of this takes time, and that means time away from the workplace. Boomers thus want to work on their own terms and schedule.

People land part-time and cyclical jobs in as many ways as there are personalities. Scaling back the hours spent at one's workplace through a phased retirement program might be an alternative, as has been shown. Or, as in the case of Louis Armstrong, a new job might develop in a serendipitous way.

Part-time work may also be home-based, as technology enables us to work from wherever we choose; this should be particularly appealing to a generation used to experimenting with new ways of doing things. About 23 million Americans work at home at least part time, the International Telework Association and Council says — and the organization expects that number to grow. In fact, according to the research and consulting firm META Group, the number of full-time telecommuters has doubled since 2000.

And then there's job hunting on the Web — investigate www.freelanceworkexchange.com or www.jobs-telecommuting.com for a look at work-at-home arrangements. Web sites that focus on part-time work include www.backdoorjobs.com, www.seniorjobbank.org and www.coolworks.com/older-bolder. Part-time opportunities are also listed at www.monster.com. And www.retiredbrains.com lists full-time, part-time and temporary jobs.

If retirement without a work focus seems bleak and working part-time or seasonally is appealing, know that with a little doing you can find such assignments. Experts predict worker shortages in health, education and technology, according to a July 2005 *Business Week* article.

CHAPTER FOUR:

NOT WORKING

And then there are those who don't find the thought of workless retirement a bleak prospect. When Jean Devero recently retired after 44 years on the job, she says, the first thing on her agenda was to "sleep for a week." Jean, like many of us, has worked very hard — every day since she was 21 years old, in fact. A single mother at a time when collecting child support was difficult — for her, impossible — she worked full time to support and raise her two children. Now, she says, she is poised to do something different, something not predicated on earning a paycheck. She is joined in her resolve to pursue some rest and relaxation by 17 percent of those surveyed by Merrill Lynch.

"Americans have become the workaholics of the industrial world," John De Graaf, the national coordinator of Take Back Your Time (www.timeday.org), says in a September 2005 article in the *Los Angeles Times*. "When you count the extra hours worked on a given day, we're on the job nine weeks more each year than most Western Europeans. The result is increased health problems, failing families, fragmented communities and a diminished life."

We are perhaps the most worn-out people on the planet. Is that some kind of badge of honor or simply stupid? Shouldn't we, at some point in our lives, take time for physical, mental and spiritual renewal? Should we live lives based on the linear model — first education, then work, then retirement, then death? Or cyclically, with breaks for rest, reflection, retooling and retraining interrupting periods of intense commitment? Both Rena Pederson in *What's Next? Women Redefining their Dreams in the Prime of Life* and Ken Dychtwald, Ph.D., in *Age Power: How the 21st Century Will Be Ruled by the New Old* say that cycling in and out of life and career modes as appropriate for the given life stage are the models of the current era.

People like Jean Devero think there might be more to life than work. "To me, retirement is a pleasant adventure into the unknown. I had always lived for the future, for a time when I would have more money to take care of my children and myself. Now I just want to live for the now," she says. "I've been remarried less than 10 years. And unlike people I know who have been married 25 years or more and want to do activities that take them away from their spouse, I want to spend time enjoying my husband; we have the time now that we aren't running from one work commitment to another. I have all the parts of my life in place — a good husband, a home, roots — and none of the insecurities of my previous days, and I just want to enjoy it all."

If you feel like Jean or are just plain tired, utilizing the retirement years for rest and recreation is a perfectly respectable, viable choice.

But when you're "ready to turn the page," as Jean puts it, when you wake up from that well-deserved nap

— what will you do? If golf is the answer, more power to you. If not, fine.

Friends and work colleagues Andy Thompson and Bob Howery both retired from executive positions at the same company a number of years ago. Now Andy is tired of retirement and has taken a new position. Bob, on the other hand, still finds satisfaction in retirement. He likes the simple pleasures of spending time with his granddaughter and working on his lake place. Each man is on the path that best suits him.

For many boomers, however, the retirement satisfaction solution might be a little different than for Bob or Andy. Instead they might choose lifelong learning or travel — or philanthropy and volunteerism.

In fact, AARP studies have shown that half of Americans over age 50 plan to incorporate community service into a retirement lifestyle. Jean is even looking at that time, although she's in no hurry. "I might like to share my experience by mentoring others at some point," she says. Whether she would do that for pay is an open question.

CHAPTER FIVE:

VOLUNTEERISM AND PHILANTHROPY

A 2002 study Peter D. Hart Research Associates conducted for Civic Ventures, a nonprofit organization encouraging older Americans to continue to be active citizens, corroborates AARP's findings. It shows that among Americans ages 50 to 75 as many as 56 percent planned to make community service part of a retired life.

For the younger members of that group, youth may have meant service in the Peace Corps or a march for a favorite cause. Today this group may still strut to the same drummer, wanting to leave the world a little bit better than it was, and desiring to bequeath some sort of legacy.

Louis Armstrong, the retired Miller Brewing executive-turned-golf-pro we met earlier, is one of them. Louis has been a male role model for Ceyvon Fields, 11, for more than three and a half years. Louis, who has lent his expertise as a member of his local Big Brothers Big Sisters board of directors for more than 10 years, took his service a step further when he applied to be a Big Brother to Little Brother Ceyvon. (Big Brothers Big Sisters' vision is to provide a mentor for every child who needs or wants one.)

"Ceyvon is bright and loaded with youthful energy that needs direction," Louis says. "We're working on distinguishing between times when it's all right to be assertive and those when it's best to back off. He's a great kid with a good heart."

In addition to tackling do-it-yourself projects and ropes courses, Armstrong and Ceyvon have been to the water park, to museums, basketball games, movies and musicals. Next on their list are church activities.

"Everything we do adds to Ceyvon's background and depth," Louis notes. "I encourage him to try things and to figure out what he can do with his many God-given talents." Not a bad contribution to make as a retiree, that encouragement.

So why does someone like Louis Armstrong devote so much time and energy to worthy causes?

"I've always been involved in community service," he says. "During my time at Miller Brewing, I was an active volunteer in my church and at the YMCA. I also led the company's United Way campaigns for five years. We set records for employee donations during that time."

But community service is not only a life habit with Louis — it's an ethos as well. "A lot of my interest in service stems from my religious training," he says. "I feel I should help out whenever and wherever God leads me."

David Burns, the retired railroad executive and community college instructor we met earlier, has another good reason for volunteering. Dave tutors at-risk students in math skills during the academic year. "I notice such a difference in my mental acuity in the summer when I don't have the stimulation of doing math with the kids," he says. His wife, Barbara, who volunteers in the prison system teaching life-control skills to inmates, also learns from her students.

Louis and David are not alone in wanting to give back to their communitics. Many of this country's retirees, sensing they are closer to the end of life than to its beginnings, want to pass on a world-changing bequest.

Carol Realini fits that bill. She's working on her legacy and doing it on a grand scale.

Carol started her career as a technologist in the mid-70s. She was good at math in school, so she pursued mathematics and computer science. During high school and early college Carol also developed an interest in social, environmental and global development issues. But she didn't see many career options in those fields, so she stuck with technology.

Carol describes her high-tech career as having had two acts. "In the first act," she says, "I worked with big companies in software and technical management. In the second, I developed four start-ups and held executive marketing and sales positions, then was CEO of two new ventures."

That time was unidimensional for Carol. She did very little except work — she read no newspapers, took no vacations and had no outside interests except family. "When my company went public in 2000, I transitioned to a board position without operational responsibilities. So I had in effect retired, and I didn't know what I would do next."

On the first day of her retirement Carol wrote a to-do list. "It seems pathetic in retrospect," she says. It read:

1. Take a walk in the woods. (Haven't done that for 10 years.)
2. Spend time with my teenagers for a change.
3. Develop friends. (I have a lot of acquaintances, but since I don't spend time with anyone, I have no close friends.)
4. Go to interesting cities and visit the sites. (I've been many places but spend all my time in hotels and office buildings.)
5. Get in shape.
6. Get a life!
7. Get to know my husband again.
8. Organize my closet; give 99 percent of business suits to a local group that helps single mothers get good jobs.
9. Go from being a human doing to a human being.

"People thought I wouldn't last a week," Carol says. "But they were wrong. After a year of travel, exercise, family and friends, I started to think about how to use my skills to do something. I didn't want another CEO position, and I definitely didn't want to work at a big company."

With time off to reflect, Carol began to revisit her other dimensions: craving adventure and exploration and loving the outdoors. She also remembered she loved the diversity of different cultures. "So when I was asked to join the board of a large NGO specializing in conflict resolution around the world, I said I would," she says.

The nongovernmental organization, Search for Common Ground (www.sfcg.org), works in the most violent places in the world to build a "capacity for peace." It uses media and community programs to create collaboration. "Their work saves lives," Carol says. "In a world where war is fashionable, they are working tirelessly to help areas traumatized by violence build lasting community."

Carol traveled to places where SFCG works, specifically to its operations in the great lakes region of Africa. The trip changed her. "Seeing homeless 5-year-olds, cities with no clean water and large areas of environmental destruction, was heart-rending. I really didn't realize these conditions existed on the scale that they do around the globe."

Carol recalls one moment in Africa — when she looked into the eyes of a child who was homeless and wearing rags. She asked the young boy if he wanted new clothes. He said no. "He told me that if he had nice clothes, people would hurt or kill him in his sleep and take his new clothes. He said instead he wanted to go to school, because, he said, 'No one can steal knowledge from you.' This boy was 7 years old. He broke my heart."

That moment, Carol recalls, was one of realization — but also connection. "I looked in his eyes and knew he was really no different from my children. He laughed like my children, he needed love, he needed to be taken care of. Only he was hungry and struggling to survive."

Carol had similar moments when she walked in the village with women who were discussing how to make their neighborhood safer for their children. "They were like me, mothers working to care for their families. Only they had so little to work with. They didn't have all the things I had come to take for granted — clean water, personal safety, education, information, human rights and small business services." Walking with these women, Carol felt a bond.

Carol returned from Africa knowing she would use her skills and resources to make things better for some of these children and their mothers. She had some decisions to make.

"Like anyone who wants to contribute, you have to decide how," she observes. "I got involved in two arenas. The first effort was to provide increased funding for 'social entrepreneurs,' local social leaders who start up and run nonprofits around the world."

Carol chose this arena for three reasons: "First, I think innovation is important to tackling global issues. Second, these talented people are making a big difference but are underfunded because most dollars go to large organizations. And finally, because these people are likely to be the future leaders of their communities, supporting them will create short- and long-term results.

My first effort takes place through the auspices of Global Giving." (www.globalgiving.com)

The second effort Carol supports is a program to use mobile phones for electronic payments. "Banking infrastructure is so weak in developing countries. People have no banking services and no payment cards. They stand in line to pay utility bills and have to pay cash for everything, often paying high fees for money orders and remittances. Yet mobile phones are everywhere and people with prepaid mobile phones are loading value in the form of minutes." As a result of her travels Carol saw a way to use prepaid mobile phones as electronic wallets, making the value loaded on the phone as fungible as cash. "I decided this had so much potential that I started another company," she says.

Carol is a different person today. She has left her job to find her work. "I've made the transition from my single-dimensional self. Today I always read the paper and make an effort to remain connected to what's happening in the world. My new venture is a for-profit, hard-work start-up. But it's one I believe will contribute to economic and social improvement."

Carol feels that her personal world has expanded. "But the transition was difficult. I had to pay my dues because I was doing new things."

Some of Carol's friends and family members think what she has undertaken is great. Others ask her why she wastes her time. "I think this split reflects what is happening in our society," she says. "Some people are too cynical or self-absorbed to do things for their communities or their globe. Others are afraid to even try, afraid they won't make a difference."

Carol finds it easy to make a difference. "Fifty dollars will save a child's life in Africa. We can't give up; we must work on these issues. Sometimes I panic because I'm not giving enough, but these problems are bigger than I am. I can only do the best I can. It will take lots of baby boomers, social entrepreneurs and others to make things better."

With regard to being afraid to try to make a difference, Carol believes that each of us has to decide our own tolerance for risk. "If you want to be super-safe, contribute to the Red Cross or volunteer at a food bank. If you want to support innovation, as I do, then know that you may do something that doesn't work out all the time, or end up the way you think it will."

It's also important to find your niche, Carol notes. "My thing is fostering innovation. This world needs all the innovation we have to solve some very hard problems."

We can't all make a difference on Carol's scale. But we can all do something.

If a life including volunteerism appeals to you, where can you get started pursuing it? By looking around, listening to the news, and reading the newspaper. Or contact the National Center for Charitable Statistics, a clearinghouse of data on American nonprofits. By perusing nccs.urban.org you can find out how many organizations serve your state. It shouldn't take long to connect with a cause. Below are a few of them.

The Nature Conservancy

The organization's mission is to preserve the plants, animals and natural communities that represent the diversity of life on Earth by protecting the lands and waters they need to survive.

Habitat for Humanity

This is a nonprofit, ecumenical Christian housing ministry dedicated to eliminating substandard housing and homelessness worldwide. Former President Jimmy Carter has made Habitat for Humanity a household word.

The Service Corps of Retired Executives

SCORE volunteers donate their time and business expertise to help America's entrepreneurs realize their business dreams.

The Peace Corps

Six percent of Peace Corps volunteers are over age 50, and the oldest is 82.

The New Road Map Foundation

The foundation is dedicated to lowering consumption in North America, improving its quality of life. Read *Your Money or Your Life* to get the flavor of this group and its goals.

Junior Achievement

This organization offers free enterprise and economic education to schoolchildren.

Experience Corps

Go to www.civicventures.org to learn more about this program, which places volunteer tutors age 55 and up in public schools in 14 cities. Such service may pay a stipend.

The Alzheimer's Association

The Alzheimer's Association, the world leader in Alzheimer research and support, is the first and largest voluntary health organization dedicated to finding prevention methods, treatments and an eventual cure for Alzheimer's.

The Executive Service Corps

This is an association of retired businessmen and women who volunteer their time to consult with nonprofit and public service agencies.

Easter Seals

Easter Seals provides exceptional services to ensure that all people with disabilities have equal opportunity to live, learn, work and play.

The Points of Light Foundation

The Points of Light Foundation & Volunteer Center National Network engages and mobilizes millions of volunteers who are helping to solve serious social problems in thousands of communities.

Your local arts organizations

The arts in America often struggle at the edge, hampered by diminishing audiences and lack of funds. This is a prime area for making your efforts count.

Organizations like these are always on the lookout for talented help. Before you hook up with a charitable cause and become a servant leader, investigate. You may be able to find a cause that suits your schedule. Pat and Shelby Adams spend three months each summer in Santa Fe, New Mexico. Pat is a docent at the Georgia O'Keeffe Museum there. Members of the museum staff are happy to have her help during the summer months only, as that is a busy time. The arrangement is similar to the scenario we saw at Borders Books, which accommodates older workers who divide their time between winter and summer homes by offering employment at each location.

Make sure that the issues that concern your nonprofit of choice resonate with you and that you like the people involved. As a true boomer, you won't want to settle for action at the margin and without influence — your skills and sense of entitlement will require a more central, helping role. If you can't identify a cause that suits you, consider starting your own nonprofit organization. Now that's leaving a legacy!

CHAPTER SIX:

LIFELONG LEARNING

To say that Bob Boyd (not his real name), president and co-founder of a Standard and Poor's 500 energy company, enjoys hard-won financial comfort is an understatement. Still, at 55, he decided to retire and pursue an advanced degree in education; he had previously served on national and local education and work-force development commissions over the years.

As a young man, Bob never had the time or resources to hike through Europe or join the Peace Corps. He went from college graduation to a full-time job in a matter of weeks, borrowing money to buy new suits for work. So, now he chose to pursue his passion as opposed to his job.

Bob had served two terms on his city's school board while building his company. Now he wanted to give his time to bettering America's educational system. He wasn't sure how to do that, but thought he'd just dive in and find out.

Bob is not the only retiree interested in going back to school. The numbers of people getting new degrees in their 60s, 70s and 80s is soaring, Marc Freedman says in *Prime Time: How Baby Boomers Will Revolutionize Retirement and Transform America*. And *Newsweek* called it a "golden age on campus."

You don't have to be seeking an advanced degree, however, to be a part of the lifelong learning movement. For some boomers, particularly those who want to start businesses or new careers after their "official" retirement, retraining may be a need. While that may necessitate getting another degree or even an advanced degree, it can also mean just taking a few brush-up courses. Many such courses of study are available, including online options. Eckerd College in St. Petersburg, Florida, and Adelphi University in Garden City, New York, even offer credit for on-the-job experience.

And then some people just want to learn for learning's sake. They are not seeking formal degrees, just the fun of study. For them, colleges and universities offer lots of one-time-only classes. These address every conceivable interest a retiree could have. For example, the *Fort Worth Star-Telegram* publishes a quarterly special section "for adults 45 and better." A May 2005 issue described local university enrichment courses, including those on language, fitness, writing, financial planning, gardening and community service.

For those who want to learn for the sheer joy of it, a Lifelong Learning Institute may be the answer. These LLIs — more than 400 of them are located mainly on college campuses nationwide — are autonomous community-based organizations dedicated to addressing the educational interests of their members, generally people of retirement age. Most LLIs offer noncredit academic programs developed by their members. Membership in most LLIs is open to anyone over age 50 regardless of previous schooling, and classes generally require no grades and no tests. LLI members frequently lead some of the academic coursework.

In 1988, Elderhostel Inc., a Boston-based nonprofit organization providing educational travel for older adults, joined with the LLIs that were then up and running to form a voluntary association known as the Elderhostel Institute Network. The organizations work together to improve the variety and quality of adult higher education. The network promotes communication between LLIs and fosters the growth of new ones. More than 4,000 courses are offered each term through America's LLIs. For more information, go to www.elderhostel.org/ein/intro.asp or e-mail network@elderhostel.org.

You can even live where you learn. Academy Village, located on 168 acres associated with the University of Arizona, is an adult residential community near Tucson, Arizona. At the center of life at Academy Village is the Arizona Senior Academy, a nonprofit organization dedicated to lifelong learning. The academy, founded by Henry Koffler, Ph.D., president emeritus of the University of Arizona, offers all residents of Academy Village a variety of educational and cultural programs. These include seminars, programs and concerts as well as panel discussions and five- to ten-week courses. A monthly fee that residents pay supports the academy's events.

Bob Buford outlines other ways to participate in lifelong learning in *Halftime: Changing Your Game Plan from Success to Significance*. These are the less formal educational tools: wide-ranging reading, listening to books on tape and enjoying a variety of media like National Public Radio. He also recommends attending conferences — as opposed to or in addition to college classes.

Whether it's something as serious as an advanced degree or as simple as exploring an interest through a short course or a good book, educational options in retirement are rich. And all it may take to get started is a visit to the online search engine Google (www.google.com). Try amazon.com for books or have a look at the Learning Annex (www.learningannex.com) for courses on personal growth.

CHAPTER SEVEN:

TRAVEL

In a recent online chat at travelwriters.com, a participant said that within ten years the over-50 crowd in the United Kingdom might well outnumber the 20-somethings in taking adventure tours and doing volunteer work abroad. The top five destinations for volunteer work were, the chat participant said, India, Ecuador, Sri Lanka, Vietnam and Peru. The top-rated projects were teaching English, conservation, community development, sports coaching and home building.

Another participant then signed in to say that she and her husband — they were nearly 60 and 76 respectively — would soon embark on a birding tour to Uganda. They would follow that with a trek to Rwanda to see mountain gorillas. "Never say 'no' until you're dead," she said.

Increasingly, baby boomers are heading out to see the world. They may have nursed a beer on the Via Veneto as youths. Now they want to do more of the same. Many of them also exhibit a philanthropic spirit not unlike that of Louis Armstrong, combining international volunteerism with travel for its own sake.

Margot Taylor, a native of the Big Apple, explains why travel is so important to her. "A few years ago I had lots of responsibilities — work, kids and my elderly mother to take care of. I felt harried. Now a lot of those obligations are behind me. So I'm free to pick up where I left off in my younger days, seeing the world and having some adventures. And I only have so many years left to see all the places I want to see, so I'm off on an excursion every chance I get."

Margot and her husband, John, make frequent trips to Europe together. But they also make journeys on their own. Margot is considering participating in a humanitarian mission to Guatemala. "It will allow me to give back to a world which has given me so much," she says, "but it also offers me something — a chance to hone my Spanish-language skills." When Margot is off on one her expeditions, John may make one of his frequent treks to Nepal or Sikim.

Jane Hardwick, a retirement coach we'll meet again later, can do her work virtually anywhere. Because her career offers this flexibility, she and her husband, a doctor, are discussing the idea of spending part of their retirement years in a recreational vehicle and on the road. Jane would pursue her coaching practice, and her husband could work locum tenens, as a temporary substitute for doctors on leave, at any chosen location. The Hardwicks could see the world and work as well. There are many ways to skin the cat.

If travel is on your list of retirement goals, finding the perfect trip is easy. Check the Sunday newspaper travel section, surf the Web or see a travel agent.

Women may want to investigate Gutsy Women Travel (www.gutsywomentravel.com), a division of

Maupintour, one of the best-known and oldest travel companies. Gutsy Women caters to women age 30 to 62 seeking to recharge in the company of like-minded others. Another option is Senior Women's Travel (www.poshnosh.com), targeting women age 50 and over. Boomer women's penchant for travel may stem from their more active lifestyles relative to their parents, according to an April 2005 *USA Today* travel article.

And speaking of being physically active, Walking the World offers "outdoor adventures for people 50 and better." On a September 2005 trip to Spain, participants walked 98 miles along the Camino de Santiago, a religious pilgrimage route for hundreds of years. Hikers like Esta Marie and Sandy Stover polished off the trails easily. Retired in Key West, Florida, the Stovers are active people. Esta Marie, a former school principal, works at a gallery one day a week and teaches English as a second language. Sandy is a writing coach at a community college and works one day a week at the front desk of a time-share.

Also consider organizations like the Earthwatch Institute (www.earthwatch.org), which engages people worldwide in scientific field research and education to promote the understanding and action necessary for a sustainable environment. Earthwatch volunteers who work on the institute's global expeditions pay a share of expedition expenses. The money they contribute to participate in an expedition is tax-deductible for American volunteers. About 35 percent of Earthwatch volunteers are 50 and older.

Another arm of Elderhostel is worth exploring. Unlike LLIs, which are local and community-based classes to which attendees commute, Elderhostel education/travel programs are short-term residential programs typically run by educational and cultural institutions. Such programs may be available in the United States or abroad and range from five to six nights in the United States and two to four weeks overseas.

Elderhostel has also launched a travel/study program initiative called Road Scholar (www.roadscholar.org). The program, led by resident experts and offered to groups of no more than 23 people, is designed to accommodate the preferences and interests of baby boomers. It offers learning and travel opportunities for those who see travel as a means of discovery. Participants take an active, hands-on role and enjoy behind-the-scenes experiences and off-the-beaten-path locations not otherwise accessible to them. Each program provides free time for self-directed learning.

Retiring in an activist manner, instead of slowly disintegrating on the golf course at your age-segregated retirement enclave, is a matter of getting your groove back — and keeping it. Planning an adventure, pushing the envelope and moving out of your comfort zone are important ingredients in keeping your old age young. Did you once dream you were the next Indiana Jones? Go out and be him while you still have time.

CHAPTER EIGHT:

THE SABBATICAL

Working like a dog, coming in under budget, dodging office politics. Running errands on your lunch hour, shuttling the kids, grooming the dog, mowing the lawn, worrying about your elderly parents. Sometimes the obligations get to be just too much. Lots of times they're too much. What if you could take a break from the stress, recharge your batteries and redefine your priorities?

Enter the sabbatical.

Isn't that just for professors? Not anymore. From personal service firms to corporations to nonprofits, extended-leave policies are burgeoning, the Society for Human Resource Management says. In conducting a June 2003 survey the society learned that 19 percent of the 584 firms polled offered unpaid sabbatical leave in 2003. That's up from 17 percent in 2002. The survey found that 6 percent of the organizations offered paid leaves of absence.

The trend is catching on. Companies like Arrow Electronics, Xerox and the commercial real estate firm Spectrum Properties offer sabbaticals, as do others. And The Merrill Lynch New Retirement Survey indicates that boomers will welcome them; the study showed that respondents would prefer cyclical periods of sabbatical over traditional retirement.

But I couldn't allow myself to do that, you say. It's true. "Many people's self-image is so tied up in work that they can't give themselves permission to pursue their dreams," says Joan DiFuria, a psychotherapist at the Money, Meaning and Choices Institute, which helps people find balance among time and money, self, relationships, work and community.

But that is precisely what many boomers are cautioning against: forfeiting the chance for deeper self-knowledge. With their interest in self-reinvention they lead the way, just as they did when they marched against the war in Vietnam. "So while most people will need to get back to work after a sabbatical to feel productive, the time they've taken off helps them find themselves and better manage the balance between work and life," says Stephen Goldbart, Ph.D., also of the institute.

Doug Dickinson, the spouse of our cyclical consultant Donna, counts among the blessings of his job a generous sabbatical program. He works for a major semiconductor company with headquarters in the San Francisco Bay Area.

The company's policy is to offer exempt (salaried) employees a six-week sabbatical with full pay in the first year after every five years on the job. Nonexempt (hourly) employees get four-week sabbaticals. In addition, exempt employees can attach two additional weeks of regular vacation time to their sabbatical for a total of eight weeks off. Nonexempt workers may add one week of vacation to their four-week sabbatical, for a total of five weeks off. Doug, an exempt employee, enjoyed his first sabbatical in 2001 and is due for another in 2006.

"In 2001," Doug says, "Donna and I went to England, France and Italy for six weeks. For someone who had never had more than three weeks' vacation in my life, six weeks felt like an eternity. By the end of the sabbatical, my race-around body had slowed to the point where I could sit in the Piazza Navona in Rome and people-watch for hours without getting bored."

Then Doug came home. "Coming back to work is the hard part," he says. "You spend the whole first week answering everyone's question: 'What did you do on your sabbatical?' Then you start to deal with the little problems that cropped up while you were gone and it's probably more irritating than normal."

Doug and Donna are already considering what to do during his upcoming sabbatical. "I'm like a kid in a candy store as far as my next sabbatical is concerned," he says. "I want to do everything. We're considering a car or train trip around the United States and Canada."

He continues: "On my first sabbatical, we rented a car in England and again in Paris to drive to Pisa. I realized I was driving 80 miles per hour on the freeways for two weeks. There was just too much to see and I couldn't slow down long enough to really see anything well. As a consequence, we blasted through England and France. We finally slowed down when we got to Sicily."

Doug doesn't think he's atypical when he says he views the sabbatical as a fantastic benefit of his job. "That and the profit-sharing program make it attractive.

There is very little turnover at my company. Unlike many high-tech companies, we have a lot of older workers." Doug sees people still working at his compny well into their retirement years. It may just be that the sabbatical and profit sharing are keeping these people around. "They're making good money and getting a chance to rest once in a while as well," he says.

"My sabbatical impacted my priorities," Doug says. "Keeping this job that lets me be so footloose every five years is important. This is the longest I have ever been with one company since I started working. Some days I feel like I could keep this up another ten years, which would put me at 68 years old."

Doug seems to be saying that the opportunity to cycle from work to rest and relaxation and back again — under the cyclical, not the linear, model — provides an incentive to stay on the job well past the time most employees would consider leaving. His company, and others like it, may be on to something that's as good for business as it is for employee well-being.

PART TWO:

RESOURCES FOR MAKING THE DECISION

CHAPTER NINE:

THINKING IT THROUGH

The first half of our lives is frenetic and noisy, as Bob Buford says in *Halftime: Changing Your Game Plan from Success to Significance*. There is little time for taking stock, for assessing what we want next. Sedlar and Miners agree in *Don't Retire, Rewire: Five Steps to Fulfilling Work That Fuels Your Passion, Suits Your Personality, or Fills Your Pocket*. The authors say busyness during this time precludes planning for future fulfillment. But that doesn't mean we shouldn't carve out time, however difficult that may be, for reflection about our upcoming activities and happiness.

In reading this book, you've looked at a variety of lifestyle choices and how they can play out in real time. Still, maybe you feel no closer to choosing the one that is right. You need a system to help you decide. Where to get that assistance? Read on. The second half comes all too soon.

CHAPTER TEN:

RETREATS

Mike and Sharon McGee of Houston enjoy their work but are nonetheless considering retirement. Still, they don't want to "just stop," Sharon says. Rather, they would like to redirect their energies. The questions are: How and where?

Fill in the blank: "When I retire I want to____." Whether the words that come to mind are "learn to cook," "start a new business" or "write the great American novel," it might make sense first to learn how to be good at retirement itself. After all, what if you retire to take up the guitar, a lifelong dream, and then discover you hate playing guitar? Wouldn't it be wise to try your notion of retirement on for size first, to give it the proverbial test drive?

A course out there helps with the visioning, and it's in a beautiful spot: Asheville, North Carolina. The course offers two weekend programs with a sampling of retirement issues at the wooded 256-acre hilltop campus of the University of North Carolina at Asheville.

The North Carolina Center for Creative Retirement, a lifelong learning, leadership and community service program, offers Paths to a Creative Retirement in Uncertain Times in two three-day workshops, generally in March and September. Through lectures, case studies and small-group discussions, the course helps people six months to five years away from retirement with unknowns related to the transition. Participants assess their ability to deal with change and the accuracy of their image of retirement, among other things.

"We suggest people explore areas they feel might become avocations before they retire, try out their fantasies, do some field testing," says Ron Manheimer, executive director of the center for 17 years. "That's better than having a dream until you retire and then finding it doesn't suit you after all."

Every Memorial Day weekend, the center also hosts a Creative Retirement Exploration Weekend, introducing the area to people considering relocating to western North Carolina — about 150 people come from more than 26 states. The weekender includes an optional Friday course, Weekend Warm Up, focusing on the social and personal implications of the retirement transition. A Monday extension, Weekend Afterglow, offers a further look at Asheville and its environs.

Ron Manheimer is extremely proud of a program that allows people like Mike and Sharon to get off the merry-go-round and contemplate life's next steps before taking them. "When was the last time you had an opportunity to stop and rethink what you want to do with your life?" he asks. "Maybe not since you graduated from college." Mike and Sharon McGee concur.

As the Asheville experience shows, not only is it a good idea to try the concept of retirement on for size. Giving some thought to the where of retirement makes sense as well. Other programs, one of them in Mississippi, can help with that end of retirement exploration.

Diana O'Toole is program manager for Hometown Mississippi Retirement, a division of the Mississippi Development Authority. She hosts Mississippi Roundabout, whose purpose is marketing and promoting 21 cities that have gone through certification. "What we've learned is that our state's smaller cities haven't been able to compete in bringing in retirees, nor could they host groups. So we designed Mississippi Roundabout, where we bring in about 15 retiring couples per trip for a look at what we have to offer. We showcase about five of our cities at a time, including the smaller ones, by taking potential retirees on a guided motor coach tour, with hotel accommodations and meals included. They get the opportunity to see if the place is a fit."

To learn more about retirement in Mississippi, go to www.visitmississippi.org/retire. To learn more about the North Carolina Center for Creative Retirement, go to unca.edu/ncccr.

CHAPTER ELEVEN:

COACHES

The busy executive dreams of the day he'll retire and finally have time for outside interests. But when he does retire he's lost. With so much time on his hands, he's baffled as to how to use it meaningfully. He needs help rethinking the work/not work issue, redirecting energies, defining retirement and reinventing his life. He needs avocational counseling — as Ken Dychtwald, Ph.D., calls it in *Age Wave: How the Most Important Trend of Our Time Will Change Your Future* — just as he may have needed vocational counseling at the height of his career. What to do?

Maybe it's time to call in a coach, the executive reasons. After all, a business coach helped him manage his career. His career coach listened to him carefully, identifying expressed objectives for which the coach held him accountable. Why not a coach to help him manage what comes next and to advise him, so that his second half is intentional, not random? Is there such a thing?

There is. Not only does retirement coaching exist as a subspecialty of the coaching business, but the niche is growing. Retirement Options, (www.retirementoptions.com) a company that teaches and certifies retirement coaches, has trained more than 500 people worldwide in the last three years. "That's a 250 percent increase in coaches trained," says Justin Johnson, the managing director. "And this year we expect more than 100 percent growth."

So what is coaching? Coaching is a supportive, confidential, peer-to-peer process that occurs between coach and client. A client may have questions such as "What is next for me in my pursuit of a fulfilling life?" or "How do I create a life adventure of my own design that expresses who I am?" A professional coach helps a client expand self-awareness about his desires, needs and values. The coach then guides the client toward the realization of life goals that the client identified through gentle nudging and the expectation of performance toward meeting those goals. Good coaching can be a gratifying experience.

Still, coaching, as with many new business and life management tools that morph into consultancies, is unlicensed and unregulated. Because the industry is in its youth, it is still ironing out legal and ethical issues. Prospective clients should thus vet prospective coaches' training, credentials and experience. And a good coach should help his clients identify very specific goals for which they are willing to be held responsible.

Where to get help? Phyllis Arnold is head of the Philly Group (www.coachphilly.com). She works with people in transition. Jane Hardwick is the CEO of Jane Hardwick Personal and Professional Coaching (www.GettingYouToGreat.com). Jane offers six-session retirement planning teleclasses, among other services. Lee Smith, Ph.D., who collaborated with Rena Pederson on *What's Next? Women Redefining Their Dreams in the Prime of Life*, is an executive coach. She also coaches people entering what she calls "Act Two." Lee's Web site is www.coachworks.com. Coaches Alexandra Mezey (www.lifeclaritycoaching.com) and Richard Haid (www.adultmentor.com) coach new and about-to-be retirees. Mezey works with people moving into what she terms "second adulthood." For Haid the term is "third quarter of life." Jeri Sedlar and Rick Miners, authors of *Don't Retire, Rewire: Five Steps to Fulfilling Work That Fuels Your Passion, Suits Your Personality, or Fills Your Pocket*, have counseled those going through the stages of career development at midlife. Now they advise boomers who want to discover personal motivations as they plan what follows official work.

What will your coach do to head you down the road to self-discovery? "A good coach helps you design your retirement mission statement," Jane Hardwick says. "If you don't already have a life mission statement, a coach will help you draft one. If you do have one, a coach helps you draft a new one, noting the differences in the two. Everything you do should contribute to that mission, and it should take into account the changes in your lifestyle. You want a life that is pleasurable, engaging and meaningful, not just busy."

And like the folks at the North Carolina Center for Creative Retirement, Jane is ever aware of the gaps between expectations and present behavior. "It's true," she says. Don't assume you'll love playing guitar in retirement if you don't own or play one now."

The International Coach Federation (coachfederation.org) offers a coaching referral service that matches clients to coaches. Clients who post their needs on the organization's Web site can then select from among coaches someone whose skills are a match for their requirements. Jeanne Bongo, the organization's coach referral service administrator, says that out of 4,245 coaches worldwide listed on her referral database, 62 cite retirement coaching as a specialty. That's not a large number — not so far. But as we've seen, the subspecialty is growing. And you only need one!

CHAPTER TWELVE:

SELF-HELP GROUPS

Don't want to hire a coach? How about joining a self-help group?

Consider, for instance, The Transition Network (www.thetransitionnetwork.org), a New York City-based, 800-member group offering guidance during this new life phase. Its peer groups (usually eight to twelve members) provide a more intimate setting for discussing life issues and meet regularly to discuss such retirement issues as time management, volunteering and finance. The network also offers lectures on career change. To date, The Transition Network has twenty-five active groups.

In her book *Retire Smart, Retire Happy: Finding Your True Path in Life,* Nancy K. Schlossberg, Ed.D., describes another self-help organization, The Retirement Group. The group is composed of retired women who meet monthly to explore their reactions to their new lifestyles.

Another such group is WomanSage (www.womansage.com) based in Orange County, California, whose mission is to empower, educate and foster mentoring relationships among mature women. The organization hosts monthly salon meetings. It also offers a quarterly journal, small special-interest groups and annual conferences.

And consider an idea from James V. Gambone, Ph.D., an expert on aging and intergenerational relationships whom we'll meet again later. He calls retirement "ReFirement®" and suggests that we form self-help groups based on the principles he's espoused in his book.

You can find support groups or form your own. To find support groups, go to civicventures.org and investigate The Next Chapter for a state-by-state links to libraries, community centers, colleges and other organizations that serve as resources for retirees. Forming your own group can be as simple as contacting friends and colleagues in your community and inviting them for coffee and discussion.

CHAPTER THIRTEEN:

COMPANY-SPONSORED PRE-RETIREMENT WORKSHOPS

Sometimes you can get help plotting your next moves while at your pre-retirement workplace and still on the job. A number of companies offer pre-retirement workshops, Gene Stone says in an article in the June 2004 issue of LOMA's *Resource*, the magazine for insurance and financial services management.

Jefferson Pilot Financial is one. It offers a Retirement Readiness Workshop over two days, Stone says. Participants complete a Retirement Success Profile highlighting 15 factors, both psychological and financial, that contribute to a successful retirement. The process compares future retirees' attitudes toward retirement with current behavior to show gaps between the two. Stone cites an example in his article of the future retiree who has pledged to a new life of woodworking but who, it turns out, doesn't even own any woodworking equipment. That's a gap that needs to be closed. Thus a company whose primary mission is financial provides good psychological advice to its employees.

For a number of years, the Evangelical Lutheran Church in America's Board of Pensions and its Vocation and Education program unit have co-sponsored pre-retirement workshops. These forums, lasting two to three days, help participants think about retirement income and individual readiness for change.

The group's current program features the aforementioned James V. Gambone, Ph.D., author of *ReFirement: A Guide to Mid-Life and Beyond.* Gambone's program focuses on the spiritual, physical and emotional aspects of retirement as well as on its vocational, intellectual and social dimensions (www.refirement.com). The sessions are open to ELCA plan members 50 and older. The sponsors offer participants two individual consultations with program representatives, and the organization says it encourages spouses to attend.

The University of Southern California also offers pre-retirement workshops, says Janette Brown, Ed.D., executive director of the university's Emeriti Center. These run alongside efforts, such as an ongoing lecture program, to keep employees connected with the university in retirement.

And Sabre Holdings offers retirement planning sessions through an agreement with Fidelity Investments, says Mike Haefner, senior vice president for human resources. The sessions consider both financial and nonfinancial aspects of retirement, such as health considerations, and encourage retiree self-accountability.

CHAPTER FOURTEEN:

FINAL THOUGHTS

As they say, there are lots of ways to skin a cat. Whether you choose to retire into continued work, full- or part-time, or to give back through philanthropy, seek another education or simply enjoy life, give yourself permission to think through the options carefully. After all, the Merrill Lynch retirement survey cited in earlier chapters found that those who took time to plan felt more confident that they would have a fulfilling retirement. It might even make sense to build enjoyable retirement activities into your pre-retirement lifestyle now — before officially leaving your workplace. That way they'll be there when your time is your own.

When you're ready, segue at your own pace from one lifestyle to the next. The way your neighbors choose to retire may work for them, but may not for you. There is no one method by which you should retire. Seek your way of retiring and take your time setting it up.

Consider the pre-retirement interests and skills you plan to build on in retirement. Decide whether your proposed next steps fit your temperament, For example, if you think you want to be an entrepreneur in Act Two, ask yourself first, "Does entrepreneurship suit my personality?" It might not.

Give equal attention to the aspects of your pre-retirement life that you'll choose to jettison. Then do more of what you like and less of what you don't like. Embrace that which energizes you, and abandon that which dampens you. After all, you've put up with energy-sapping traits in others and draining situations and behaviors all your adult life. Spurn them now.

Define success loosely. You might preclude some terrific adventures if you don't. And don't be too linear or rational in the planning; that can be limiting.

Seek balance. Remaining active ensures a youthful outlook, but make time for an inner, mindful, spiritual life as well. God knows, you were too busy for that in younger years.

Coordinate your idea of retirement with that of your spouse. That will help avoid unpleasant surprises and opposed expectations.

And remember that transitions take emotional energy and that disengaging from the old and adjusting to the new take time. You are exiting roles you have played for a long time, and new roles may feel strange at first.

For men this may be particularly difficult. Women generally move from one phase to another throughout their lives; career may be followed by the jolt of new motherhood, a return to work, which is followed by the empty nest, then retirement. Men generally work straight through, with fewer periods off to concentrate on child-rearing and to experience the emptiness when it ends. For them retirement may be the biggest or only jolt they experience. Women may better accept this newest of numerous life changes. Women often pursue in midlife a passion deferred while juggling a career and family and child-rearing responsibilities, according to a May 2005 *Time* magazine article on the female midlife crisis.

Periods of grieving and confusion might ensue during this time of adjustment and option selection. False starts are also OK; if you try one of the lifestyles and it doesn't suit you, simply head in a new direction using what you've learned to make a better choice the next time.

Finally, abandon all self-talk about being too old to start over. No self-respecting baby boomer does that.

It's all right to search, explore. That's what this book and this time — your time — is for, after all.

Go ahead. Live a life that's different from Dad's if you choose to. Play golf, or walk away from the course and back to school. Work as much or as little as you choose to, or not at all. Leave a legacy or write a memoir. You've paid your dues. Reward yourself by living your own authentic life!

SUGGESTED READING

Buford, Bob. *Finishing Well.* Nashville: Integrity Publishers, 2004.

Buford, Bob. *Halftime: Changing Your Game Plan from Success to Significance.* Grand Rapids: Zondervan 1994.

Cohen, Gene D., M.D., Ph.D. *The Creative Age: Awakening Human Potential in the Second Half of Life.* New York: Harper Collins, 2001.

Dychtwald, Ken, Ph.D. *Age Power: How the 21st Century Will Be Ruled by the New Old.* New York: Tarcher/Putnam, 2000.

Dychtwald, Ken, Ph.D. *Age Wave: How the Most Important Trend of Our Time Will Change Your Future.* New York: Bantam Doubleday, 1990.

Dychtwald, Ken, Ph.D. *The Power Years: A User's Guide to the Rest of Your Life.* Hoboken: John Wiley & Sons Inc., 2005.

Freedman, Marc. *Prime Time: How Baby Boomers Will Revolutionize Retirement and Transform America.* New York: Public Affairs, Perseus Books Group, 1999.

Friedan, Betty. *The Fountain of Age*. New York: Simon and Schuster, 1993.

Gambone, James V. *ReFirement: A Guide to Mid-Life and Beyond*. Minneapolis: Kirk House Publishers, 2000.

Miners, Rick and Sedlar, Jeri. *Don't Retire, Rewire: Five Steps to Fulfilling Work That Fuels Your Passion, Suits Your Personality, or Fills Your Pocket*. Alpha Books: Indianapolis, 2003.

Pederson, Rena with R. Lee Smith. *What's Next? Women Redefining Their Dreams in the Prime of Life*. New York: Perigee Books, 2001.

Roszak, Theodore. *America the Wise: The Longevity Revolution and the True Wealth of Nations*. Boston and New York: Houghton Mifflin Company, 1998.

Saussy, Carroll. *The Art of Growing Old: A Guide to Faithful Aging*. Minneapolis: Augsburg Books, 1998.

Schlossberg, Nancy K. *Retire Smart, Retire Happy: Finding Your True Path in Life*. Washington, D.C.: APA Life Tools, 2004.

Stone, Howard and Stone, Marika C. *Too Young to Retire: 101 Ways to Start the Rest of Your Life*. New York: Plume, 2004.

ABOUT THE AUTHOR

Joan Fitting Scott is an award-winning freelance writer specializing in baby boomer issues. She has written for *Senior News* and is a regular contributor to *Senior Voice.*

NOTES

NOTES

NOTES

NOTES

NOTES

NOTES

NOTES

NOTES

NOTES